Yoga and Diet: The Mindful Connection

Also by Gunn Helene Arsky:

For children:
Rikka og næringsstoffene

Non-fiction:
Liten ernæringslære
Helgefri slanking
Barn & diabetes
Kostskolen. 555 spørsmål og svar om mat, helse og trening
Spis deg ung
Maten barna elsker å hate

eBook:
Yoga and Diet: The Mindful Connection

Co-author:
Liv og helse
Takk for mat
Mat- og helseboka
Litt lettere
7 slankekurer som garantert virker
Spis deg frisk fra A til Å
Barnehageboken
Kosthåndboken
Helsestasjonsboka
Ernæring – mer enn mat og drikke

Yoga and Diet: The Mindful Connection

GUNN HELENE ARSKY

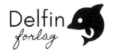

© Delfin forlag, Halden, Norway 2020

ISBN 978-82-692036-1-5

1. edition 2020

Cover design: Gunn Helene Arsky
Cover photo: unsplash.com/@creatveight
Author photo: Veronika van Groningen
Typesetter: Gunn Helene Arsky
Print: Amazon.com 2020

www.gunnhelenearsky.no

To Juha, we did it!

DISCLAIMER

You should consult your physician or other health care professional before changing your diet to determine if it is right for your needs. This book offers health and nutritional information and is designed for educational purposes only. You should not rely on this information as a substitute for, nor does it replace, professional medical advice, diagnosis, or treatment. If you have any concerns or questions about your health, you should always consult with a physician or other health care professional.

Do not disregard, avoid or delay obtaining medical or health related advice from your health care professional because of something you may have read in this book. The use of any information provided in this book is solely at your own risk.

MY FREE GIFT TO YOU

I am so happy that you bought my book – thank you very much! I would like to offer you this free gift – my eBook with healthy and tasty recipes for a greener, more plant-based life.

Here's the download url:

https://gunnhelenearsky.no/wp-content/uploads/2020/10/eBook-recipes-Gunn-Helene-Arsky.pdf

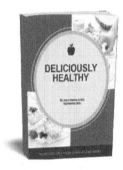

INTRODUCTION

This book is what I was in desperate need of, but didn't have, when I started out as a yoga practitioner in 2005. And here it is – a guide to the mindful connection between your yoga practice on the mat, and your diet off the mat.

- What happens when we connect the ancient *Yoga Sutras* of Patanjali with modern nutritional science?
- Or when mindful eating meets *Chakra* foods?
- Or when we address the *Ayurvedic* dietary advice for each of our body and mind types, when we know what the *Hatha Yoga Pradipika* has to say about food and diet?

Answer: We get to understand why our bodies start craving other types of food when we engage deeply in our yoga practice.

This book is a gift to all of you devout yoga students and experienced yoga teachers out there.

When I first encountered yoga, I perceived it solely as a form of exercise. And I loved it! Feeling my body getting stronger and more supple from week to week, and mastering progressively more challenging poses. I started noticing all parts of my body in a new way. I also noticed my energy levels like never before. And as time passed and I got more and more attuned to the subtleties of yoga, energetic work, and bodily awareness, I could hear my body asking for a shift. A shift in the kind of energy I fed it, no less.

Holding a Master's degree in nutritional physiology, I thought I knew all about healthy eating. But now, listening closely, I could hear my body asking for less meat. Less fish. More vegetables. More legumes. More fruits.

And when I did what my body was asking of me, I felt energized in a whole new way. I didn't need my evening nap, I didn't collapse on the couch after 9PM, I didn't feel dead tired when I woke up in the morning.

This major energy shift made me curious. And because my Yoga Teacher Training contained a lot about Patanjali's Yoga Sutras – including the *Yamas* and the concept of *Ahimsa*, I got intrigued.

- What about yoga had made me more attuned to my dietary needs?
- Was there a known connection between my yoga practice on the mat, and my dietary choices off the mat? Meaning – was this dietary change embodied in the yoga practice, and if so, where did it come from?

And that is what this book is all about.

The root connection between the foods we eat, and the yoga we practice is many thousand years old. And it is highly relevant even to this day.

I invite you to follow me on the path of understanding the connection between yoga and food, so you can create your own path in a mindful way.

TABLE OF CONTENTS

ANCIENT TEXTS AND MODERN SCIENCE

I feel that it is important to have a basic understanding of the backdrop of yoga and diet. That is why I start this journey with the beginning, some 2000 years ago. But feel free to skip around in this book, many of us find it more fruitful to follow our own logic. It is just like being on your yoga mat, actually. This is your time, and your practice. Do with it as you please.

After reading the sections in this chapter you will know how the ancient yoga texts address food and diet, and how this manifests itself today in various vegetarian diets and yoga traditions.

What is Patanjali's Yoga Sutras?

In his famous *Yoga Sutras,* Patanjali presents the Eight Limbs of Yoga, where we find the connection between yoga and the food we eat. If you haven't already read this book, I encourage you to do so.

Patanjali was a sage in India, and he is thought to be the author of a number of Sanskrit works, including the Yoga Sutras. There are no accurate records of when he lived, but he probably lived sometime between 200 BCE and 400 CE. Some sources even say that the texts attributed to Patanjali were written by several different sages bearing the same name.

The greatest of these ancient texts are the Yoga Sutras, a classical yoga text. This is a collection of 196 Indian sutras (aphorisms) on yoga. It was the most translated ancient Indian text in the medieval era. If *sutra* is an unfamiliar word to you, think about suture (from surgery), a suture means a thread, or a strand. The Yoga Sutras are short sentences – sutras – that need interpretation and elaboration to be meaningful.

The text was forgotten for nearly 700 years, from the 12th to the 19th century. The text made a comeback in the late 19th century due to the efforts of Swami Vivekananda and others. The Yoga Sutras states the first known yoga philosophy and is based on Jainism, Buddhism, and what we know as Hinduism today.

The text has four parts or *padas*:

- *Samadhi* – here you find the famous sutra: *Yogas citta-vritti-nirodhah* (yoga is the removing of the fluctuations of the mind)
- *Sadhana* (practice) – here he describes *Kriya* yoga and *Ashtanga* yoga, and this is also where we find the food
- *Vibhuti* – about yogic powers or manifestations
- *Kaivalya* – chapter on liberation

Perhaps you noticed the mention of Ashtanga yoga above? It might not be what you think. Patanjali is talking about Ashtanga yoga as the Eight Limbs of Yoga. *Asht* means eight in Sanskrit. Most of this yoga is a spiritual, not a physical, yoga practice.

Ashtanga Vinyasa Yoga, on the other hand, is very much a practice. This is a style of yoga as exercise, created by K. Pattabhi Jois during the 20th century. Confusingly, it is often called Ashtanga Yoga for short.

In the next section we will dive into a specific part of the Eight Limbs of Yoga. They have shaped our perception of the alchemy of yoga and food, and flavoured our palates.

The Power of Ahimsa

In this section we look more closely at the *Yamas* as stated by Patanjali, and specifically the first Yamas, namely *Ahimsa*. What is this, and how is it affecting our choice of foods?

"Ahimsa is the highest duty. Even if we cannot practice it in full, we must try to understand its spirit and refrain as far as is humanly possible from violence."

This is a quote by Mahatma Gandhi, India's great hero and a beacon of modest living. He recommended living by the principle of *Ahimsa* – non-violence. Gandhi got the principle from Patanjali. Because in his famous Yoga Sutras, Patanjali presents the Eight Limbs of Yoga, where we find the connection between yoga and the food we eat.

The Eight Limbs of Yoga

The goal of our physical yoga practice is to build a body that is strong enough and has enough endurance to sit through long periods of meditation. And in order to reach *samadhi* – oneness with the object of meditation – we need to have all other aspects under control first. These aspects are split into eight segments, or steps, that gradually move from the physical into the spiritual. Patanjali is very practical. He starts his eight steps with the most physical aspect, *Yamas*.

- *Yamas* - restraints or ethics of behaviour – this is the only part we will need to explore in this book
- *Niyamas* - observances
- *Asana* - physical postures
- *Pranayama* - control of the prana (breath)
- *Pratyahara* - withdrawal of the senses
- *Dharana* - concentration
- *Dhyana* - meditation
- *Samadhi* - absorption

Yamas are ethical vows in the Yogic tradition, and can be thought of as moral imperatives, rules to live by. The five Yamas listed by Patanjali are:

- *Ahimsa*: non-violence, non-harming other living beings through actions and speech. This is the key, Patanjali tells us, to maintaining both harmonious relationships in the world, and a tranquil inner life.
- *Satya*: truthfulness, non-falsehood. Seeing and reporting things as they are, rather than the way we would like them to be.
- *Asteya*: non-stealing. Intangibles, such as information and emotional favours, are more likely to be the objects stolen in our world. Try giving instead.
- *Brahmacarya*: chastity, marital fidelity or sexual restraint. The sage tells us that when the mind is freed from domination by the senses, sensual pleasures are replaced by inner joy.
- *Aparigraha*: non-greed, non-grasping, non-possessiveness. When we make good use of our possessions and enjoy them without becoming emotionally dependent on them, then they neither wield power over us, nor lead to false identities and expectations.

Why are the Yamas so important? In Sutra 2.31, Patanjali calls the Yamas *Mahavratam*, which means a great vow. Patanjali writes that practice of the Yamas is universal, and it should not be limited by class, place, time or circumstances. Meaning – they are also valid today, in our modern world.

The commentaries on the Yamas state how and why each of the self-restraints help in the personal growth of an individual. For example, in Sutra 2.35, Patanjali states that the virtue of non-violence and non-injury to others (Ahimsa) leads to the abandonment of enmity, a state that leads the yogi to the perfection of inner and outer amity with everyone, everything.

A little reminder: remember to practice non-violence towards yourself too. This may affect your food choices in another direction than you think!

How is Ahimsa affecting our choices of food?

The concept of «non-violence» could infer a bias towards vegetarianism. There is an ethical, or moral, aspect to this interpretation, but also a bodily aspect – how do you feel when you eat different kinds of foods? This is where I came from, I had a bodily experience of non-violence towards myself when I changed my diet. Many of the great yogis of our time were or still are vegetarian or vegan, and the more we reflect upon our relationship with animals around us, the more we feel united (yoga = to yoke, to unite) with nature, the more many of us wish to change our diets.

I believe that if you feel the change, you can live the change.

Hatha Yoga Pradipika

One last thing about the ancient yoga texts before we look at vegetarian diets today. After the Yoga Sutras, another major text has come to inform our yoga of today. This text is called *Hatha Yoga Pradipika* and was written by Svatmarama around year 1400 CE. Hatha yoga is the source of nearly all of the physical yoga styles we practice in the West today. This includes Iyengar yoga, Kripalu yoga, Ashtanga Vinyasa yoga, and even Restorative yoga. In India you may also find other kinds of yoga with roots in the *Bhagavad Gita* and *Upanishads: Bhakti* yoga (selfless devotion), *Jnana* yoga (knowledge or self-study), *Karma* yoga (action) and *Raja* yoga (meditation). Each type of yoga is said to offer a path to *moksha* (spiritual liberation) and self-realization. When I use the word *yoga* in this book, I mean the yoga we practice in the West – Hatha based, with breathwork, chanting and meditation.

Hatha Yoga Pradipika is divided into four chapters, covering: *Asana*, *Pranayama*, *Mudra* and *Samadhi*. The Hatha Yoga texts place major emphasis on *mitahara*, which translates to 'measured diet' or 'moderate eating'. *Mitahara* is also a concept in Indian yoga philosophy that integrates awareness about food, drinks, balanced diets, and consumption habits and its effect on one's body and mind.

Several sections of the Hatha Yoga Pradipika discuss the importance of a proper diet for the body. They link the food we eat and our eating habits to balancing the body, and gaining most benefits from the practice of physical Hatha yoga. Eating is a form of devotional act, to the temple that our body is. Mitahara is an essential part of a holistic Hatha yoga practice – also today.

Plant-based diets today

"It is my view that the vegetarian manner of living, by its purely physical effect on the human temperament, would most beneficially influence the lot of mankind."

— Albert Einstein

How I love this quote! And it is the perfect connection between the old philosophical texts and our modern way of eating.

In this section we study the different kinds of plant-based diets – from the flexitarian and pescatarian to the vegetarian and vegan diet. We also look at the scientific evidence for what positive health effects a green(er) diet may have.

But first of all, what is a plant-based diet? In short, it is a diet where most of your nutrients come from plant foods. It can be mostly or entirely plant-based, so a plant-based diet is not necessarily vegetarian. It will also look different from person to person, or from country to country.

Did you know that 26% of Millennials are vegetarians or vegans, and that 10% of the world's population follows some kind of vegetarian diet?

Humans are omnivorous – capable of consuming diverse plant and animal-derived foods. Meaning we can eat everything. Fossil evidence from wear patterns on teeth indicates that early humanoids were opportunistic omnivores, generally subsisting on a plant-based diet, but supplementing with meat and fish when possible.

So, we *can* eat everything. But *will* we eat everything?

There are so many reasons to eat plant-based. Here are some of them and some explanatory examples:

- Environmental reasons – beef production increase the CO_2 emissions
- Religious – Hindus and Buddhists are often vegetarian, Jains are always vegan
- Economic – many people around the world can't afford meat
- Moral or ethical – cruelty to animals is unavoidable in meat production
- Traditional – in areas where many are vegetarians because of religion, others may practice vegetarianism as a tradition
- Health – because your doctor ordered it, or you found out yourself

Yoga is a philosophical reason to eat plant-based, and it is based on the moral and ethics of non-violence. But philosophically inclined plant-based eaters can reap the fruits: better health and environmental benefits.

The Flexitarian Diet

This diet or lifestyle encourages mostly plant-based foods, while allowing meat and other animal products in moderation. It is more flexible than fully vegetarian or vegan diets, and hence it is easier to indulge in a variety of foods in social settings. You can have that meat stew your grandmother cooked for you without any feelings of guilt. If you're looking to add more plant foods to your diet but don't want to completely cut out meat, going flexitarian may be for you.

Here are some tips on the way to becoming a true flexitarian:

- Eat mostly fruits, vegetables, legumes and whole grains.
- Focus on protein from plants instead of animals.
- Be flexible and incorporate meat and animal products from time to time.
- Eat the least processed, most natural form of foods.
- Limit added salt, sugar, and sweets.

This way of eating has become increasingly popular, also because of the environmental benefits. The major breakthrough for this way of eating is perhaps the Meat Free Mondays, a clear sign that even meat lovers love a green day each week.

The Pescatarian Diet

A pescatarian is someone who chooses to eat a vegetarian diet, but who also eats fish and/or other seafood. It is mainly a plant-based diet consisting of whole grains, nuts, legumes, and healthy fats, with fish and seafood playing a significant role as a main protein source. Many adhere to this kind of diet in order to reap the health benefits of a plant-based diet, plus heart-healthy fish. Others choose this way of eating to curb the environmental impact of their diet. And others simply choose this as a matter of taste.

The Vegetarian Diet

According to the Vegetarian Society, a vegetarian is someone who does not eat any meat, poultry, game, fish, shellfish or by-products of animal slaughter. But other than that, the vegetarian diets may vary a lot.

Vegetarian diets contain various amounts of fruits, berries, vegetables, grains, legumes, nuts and seeds. The inclusion of dairy and eggs depends on the type of diet you follow.

The most common types of vegetarians include:

- **Lacto-ovo vegetarians:** Vegetarians who avoid all animal flesh, but do consume dairy and egg products.
- **Lacto vegetarians:** Vegetarians who avoid animal flesh and eggs, but do consume dairy products.
- **Ovo vegetarians:** Vegetarians who avoid all animal products except eggs.

The Vegan Diet

A vegan diet can be viewed as the strictest form of vegetarianism. Veganism is currently defined by the Vegan Society as *"a way of living that attempts to exclude all forms of animal exploitation and cruelty as much as possible."* This also includes exploitation for food and any other purpose, like leather shoes or belts, or circus animals, or animal experiments.

Vegans believe that animals have a right to be free from human use. Therefore, a vegan diet not only excludes animal flesh, but also dairy, eggs and animal-derived ingredients. These include gelatine (gelling agent), honey, carmine (red colour often used in cosmetics and foods), casein, albumin and whey (milk proteins in protein powder), and some forms of vitamin D3.

Health benefits of a plant-based diet

A plant-based diet is often touted as the healthiest approach to eating, and its benefits extend way beyond weight loss. On the next pages you will find an assortment of the major health benefits and their underlying mechanisms.

Prevent heart disease because of better cholesterol levels

A high cholesterol level increases your risk of various types of heart disease. Cholesterol forms in your body when you eat fats – especially when you consume saturated fat from butter, cheese, bacon, egg yolks, and fatty meats. Cutting out those foods will reduce your own production of cholesterol.

But animal produce also contains cholesterol. So there's a double whammy when reducing the intake of these kinds of foods.

In addition, plant foods contain bioactive substances that will protect your cholesterol from turning rancid (getting oxidized). Oxidized cholesterol is especially bad for your heart and blood vessels. Should we call this a triple whammy, perhaps?

Lower blood pressure and less risk of stroke

A diet rich in vegetables and fruits is high in potassium. This mineral takes part in regulating the fluid levels inside and outside all our cells. It helps us release excess water, and hence our blood pressure normalises.

Cooking from scratch (as many will have to do when following a plant-based diet) also means less salt used. This also lowers our blood pressure. A lower blood pressure in turn puts less pressure on the blood vessels in our brain, and hence we have a lowered risk of stroke.

Prevent type 2 diabetes

Type 2 diabetes is a lifestyle disease most commonly resulting from an unbalance in energy intake and expenditure. A plant-based diet is usually lower in calories than other diets – although it definitely doesn't come automatically! But eating more vegetables high in fibres will stabilize your blood sugar levels.

Eating leaner, that is more protein-rich pulses, rather than sausages or marbled meats, will lower your intake of saturated fats. Unsaturated fats from nuts, seeds, and plant oils contain bioactive fatty acids that will lower your risk of type 2 diabetes.

And if you cut down on refined sugar, your body will need less insulin to cope with controlling the blood sugar levels. This again protects your pancreas from wearing out.

Keep a healthy weight

Major studies have shown that on average, vegetarians and vegans are slimmer than omnivores. As mentioned above, a plant-based diet is usually less calorific than a regular diet per weight unit. Say you swap your 150 gram pork chop with 150 grams of chickpeas for dinner – this will cut your energy intake in half. And snacking on fruits and berries instead of chocolate or potato chips also automatically cuts your calorie intake, without you even thinking about it. But simply cutting out meat from your diet won't do the trick, you have to increase your intake of plant foods too.

Live longer

This is a great health benefit! Studies have shown that when all other lifestyle factors are the same (e.g. smoking, physical activity, work situation etc.), those who eat vegetarian or vegan diets will live longer. This has to do with something called telomere length. A telomere is the end of your chromosomes. The shorter they are, the shorter you will live, basically.

Plant foods contain antioxidants and other bioactive substances that will protect your telomeres from shortening. Isn't that amazing?

Decrease risk of cancer

Plant foods naturally contain high levels of bioactive substances, often referred to as antioxidants. But they have many other ways of working in our bodies, than merely prevent fats from oxidizing. These bioactive substances are highly effective when it comes to battling cancer. They do their work both before cancer develops and also may help reduce the size and spread of some forms of cancer. And the best part is that studies show that powders and extracts are less beneficial than eating whole foods. I'm all for super foods, but in their natural shape and form.

Another gamechanger when choosing to eat plant-based, is that you reduce the intake of red meat and processed meats – foods that are known to increase your risk of cancer. Red meat includes pork, beef, veal, and lamb. Processed meat includes bacon, ham, lunch meats, meat jerky, hot dogs, salami, and other cured meat products.

Keep brain healthy and young

This bit is important, because what good will it do us to live long, if our brains aren't quite with us? The bioactive substances from plant foods will keep your brain cells live longer. The fats covering the 'arms' of the brain cells (the myelin sheath) will stay intact so that the electrical signals get from A to B without interruption or leakage.

If you include walnuts, linseeds, hemp seeds and chia seeds in your diet, they will provide you with ample amounts of omega-3, the essential fatty acid that will make the tiny blood vessels in your brain relax, so blood can pass freely to provide oxygen and nutrients to all the cells.

The health benefits of changing to a plant-based diet are there for you at all levels. Even going for the Meat Free Monday option will give you a slightly better health. So it is not a case of all or nothing, it is a continuum where every bit matters.

With all these benefits, and a body that is speaking to you, asking you to live the change – is it any wonder that some modern yoga traditions have internalized the plant-based diet? I think not. And in the next section we will look at how this may manifest.

Example: Jivamukti yoga and veganism

Not all styles of yoga are explicit in their approach to Ahimsa. That is why Jivamukti yoga, one of the younger Western yogic traditions, is an interesting example. Maybe you have practiced Jivamukti yoga? It is a Hatha yoga style with strong classes and much fun, often accompanied by upbeat music.

Jivamukti yoga was founded in New York City, USA, in 1984, by David Life and Sharon Gannon. They had only met the year before. Being authors, artists, musicians, and animal activists they embodied the Ahimsa concept and a plant-based lifestyle.

David Life and Sharon Gannon follow guru Swami Nirmalananda, guru Sri K. Pattabhi Jois, and guru Shri Brahmananda Sarasvati. Each of their gurus guided them further on their individual spiritual paths, and the teachings of their gurus helped shape Jivamukti yoga.

The two wanted the practice of asana to become more than a mere physical exercise to keep one's body fit, or to increase strength or flexibility. They made yoga a way to improve one's relationship to all others, with the goal of enlightenment. In this context enlightenment means the dissolution of the sense of separateness, the realization of the oneness of being, the discovery of lasting happiness.

The core philosophy of Jivamukti yoga is expressed through five tenets which form the foundation:

- Ahimsa (non-violence, veganism)
- Bhakti (devotion, intention)
- Dhyana (meditation)
- Nada (deep listening, music, speech)
- Shastra (study of yogic teachings, chanting)

The Jivamukti teachers embody these tenets, so that they colour all of his or her teachings in all types of Jivamukti classes.

In one of her blog posts, Sharon Gannon writes:

I asked my first spiritual teacher, the alchemist Randy Hall, "How do I become enlightened?," and he responded, "First, learn how to cook, clean, and garden." I was disappointed, but soon saw the magic of the reply.

And so Sharon Gannon has published two books on cooking. I recommend them both:

Simple recipes for joy. A new way of living: peacefully, healthfully, and consciously. This book is filled with 200 recipes from Sharon's Jivamuktea Café and includes cruelty-free burritos, chocolate mousse, and flower salads.

She has also published *Yoga and veganism: The diet of enlightenment.* This book is more of a manifesto, and a great way to dig deeper into these matters.

Maybe you wonder: Must Jivamukti yoga teachers adhere to veganism? During the teacher training, students are shown a range of films, including some on animal rights and veganism, like Cowspiracy. These are painful to watch, and painful to discuss. Most Jivamukti yoga teachers are vegan and will promote this way of life in yoga classes.

As I mentioned in the beginning of this section, few yoga traditions are as explicit in their approach to food as Jivamukti yoga. But is there a true yogic diet? In order to answer this question we will dive into ancient Indian medicinal traditions in the next chapter.

AYURVEDA AND THE SATTVIC DIET

"When diet is wrong, medicine is of no use. When diet is right, medicine is of no need."

– Ayurvedic proverb

In this chapter you will get a basic understanding of the *Ayurvedic* principles of food and diet. After reading all the sections, you will know your body and mind type and know how to apply the principles relevant to you.

The principles and practice of Ayurveda

Yoga may inspire you to eat plant-based, but food has a central place in the traditional Indian way of preventing illness and maintaining good health. We are talking about *Ayurveda*. And maybe you have had a taste of Ayurveda already, without even knowing it?

I'm thinking of Golden Milk, or Turmeric Latte, one of the most embraced Ayurvedic remedies here in the West. I'll share my favourite recipe with you at the end of this section!

Ayurveda is a traditional medical system from India, often used to complement yoga. We will have to make do with an outline of the theories and practices here – Ayurveda is far too big of a subject to address in this concise book.

So in this section we will look at the principles for this medical system and the remedies they utilize.

The history of Ayurveda

Yoga and Ayurveda are two interrelated branches of the same tree of *Vedic* knowledge that encompasses all of human life and the entire universe. The Vedic period (1500 – 500 BCE), is the period in the late Bronze Age and early Iron Age of the history of India, when the *Vedas* (liturgical texts) were composed in the northern Indian subcontinent.

It is important to understand the respective roles of Ayurveda and yoga in the Vedic system. Yoga and Ayurveda are not merely two separate but related healing disciplines of India. Each one has its unique place and function, but they both overlap on various levels.

- Yoga – inner spiritual work
- Ayurveda – bodily medical work

Ayurveda, meaning knowledge of life and longevity, developed as a set of theoretical ideas in the mid-first millennium BCE. It shows parallels with *Samkhya* and yoga philosophy, Buddhism and Jainism. The wisdom is said to have been passed from gods to sages to human physicians.

Ayurveda emphasizes balance, and suppressing natural urges is considered unhealthy and claimed to lead to illness. For example, to suppress sneezing (like we do when we are near others) is said to potentially give rise to shoulder pain. And hence you will hear a lot of loud sneezing when you're out and about in India. However, people are also cautioned to stay within the limits of reasonable balance and measure when following nature's urges. For example, emphasis is placed on moderation of food intake, sleep, and sex.

Ayurvedic principles

Everything must find balance and order, according to Ayurveda. And illness is seen as an unbalance, or disorder. But in contrast to Western allopathic medicine, which sees an infected liver as an infected liver no matter whose body that liver resides in, Ayurveda takes this ownership into consideration.

The theory says that we are all made up of three bodily humours – the *Doshas*. These are known as *Vata*, *Pitta*, and *Kapha* Dosha. Our particular mix of the Doshas is unique, and this will inform the Ayurvedic physician when treating your infected liver.

The Doshas are made up of a combination of five elements:

1. **Ether** is the first element and is often referred to as space, or emptiness. Because ether is empty space, it is known as the element that the other elements fill. The ear and the mouth, as well as all empty spaces in our body, are associated with this element.
2. **Air** is the second element, and represents oxygen, breath, motion, and lightness. This element is present in the respiratory system and nerves.
3. **Fire** is the third of the elements and is closely associated with the eyes and the body's heat. Fire is also associated with thoughts, emotions, and obsessions.
4. **Water** is the fourth element and the protector of the body. Water is expressed in the body in five distinct ways: saliva, stomach, the nerves, the joints, and the respiratory system. It's also associated with the tongue and blood.
5. **Earth** is the last of the elements and evolves from the previous four. It also contains these elements within it. This element is heavily associated with our sense of smell, bones, nails, and teeth.

Vata Dosha is made from Ether and Air. Pitta Dosha is made from Fire and Water. And Kapha Dosha is made from Water and Earth. We will address the three Doshas in more detail later on, and you will also get to determine your Dosha.

Back to the Ayurvedic principles: An imbalance or disorder can manifest in one, or more, of our seven *dhatus* – these are tissue types, including blood, lymph, bone, and marrow. Each of the dhatus is thought to be built out of a previous one, and they develop from the nourishment that comes from the digestive system.

And finally, another central issue in Ayurveda is the *gunas*. All the qualities of the world have been identified as three basic gunas; *Tamas*, *Rajas*, and S*attva*. Inertia is called Tamas. Activity is called Rajas. Transcendence is called Sattva. These three gunas affect illness and health, but also everything in the world, from single atoms to entire galaxies.

Diagnostics

When you visit an Ayurvedic practitioner, she arrives at diagnosis through direct questioning, observation and a physical exam, as well as inference. She uses basic techniques such as taking the pulse with three fingers, thus identifying the strength of your Vata, Pitta, and Kapha pulse. She observes the shape and colour of your tongue, eyes and physical form. And she listens to the tone of your voice.

Based on this, she will give you an assessment and recommendation for your treatment – that is, your balancing. This can involve massages and herbal remedies, but will almost always involve establishing a morning routine and dietary advice.

Massage

Ayurvedic massage combines the principles of Ayurveda and pressure points. This type of massage is designed to create balance among the mind, body, and spirit, and help the body heal itself. There are two main types of massages.

Oil massage: During an Ayurvedic massage, organic oil blends are infused with Ayurvedic herbs and heated to promote relaxation and detoxification. The oils are chosen to balance your dominant Dosha. At the right temperature, these oils enter the body through the skin and pores, bind to the *ama* (toxins, in Ayurvedic tradition), and are released to detoxify the body. *Abhyanga*, *gandharva*, and *marma* massages use this technique.

Dry massage: *Garshan* massage is a traditional Ayurvedic dry massage that stimulates the skin and enhances the blood and lymphatic circulation to release accumulated toxins faster. This detox massage is given with raw silk or cotton gloves and light, rhythmic, vigorous strokes to remove dead skin layers, leaving the skin supple and glowing.

Herbal remedies

Herbs are at the very heart of the Ayurvedic tradition. Practitioners will generally use Ayurvedic herbs such as *triphala*, *guggul*, *boswellia*, and *gotu kola* to cleanse the body, boost defence against disease, and keep the mind, body, and spirit in balance. These herbs have been used for centuries to promote mental clarity, radiant skin, lustrous hair, manageable weight, healthy function of the liver, and a robust immune system, among other benefits. Several scientific studies have confirmed some of the claimed effects of the herbs.

A little note of caution: Be careful about what herbal remedies you buy. Unfortunately, many of the Indian herbal products contain heavy metals and/or are laced with drugs. This is dangerous. You may also find counterfeit products made from plants with no effect. And then you won't reap any of the benefits.

Morning routine

The Ayurvedic morning routine sets the tone for your day. The whole routine takes a while, so prepare for the first step – you have to get up early!

Get up in the small hours, preferably before 6AM, to feel light and bright. After 6 o'clock, Kapha Dosha takes over, and you will feel heavy and drowsy when getting up. Then, go to your bathroom and begin the many steps of the routine:

- Cleanse your face, mouth, and eyes

29

- Drink lukewarm water
- Sit on the toilet, preferably to urinate, as well as defecate
- Scrape your tongue with a silver spoon or tongue scraper, clean your teeth, and gargle with oil
- Use nasal and ear oils if necessary
- Give yourself an Abhyanga oil massage before bathing and dressing
- Essential oil perfume may be used
- Then do your yoga asana practice, your pranayama breathwork, and your meditation
- Breakfast!

Here is an easy and tasteful **Ayurvedic apple breakfast** recipe you can try out:

Dice one fresh, sweet apple into small pieces, without core. Place the apple pieces in a small pot, along with 5 whole cloves and 3 tablespoons of water. Place a lid on the pot and let cook until the apple pieces are soft. Discard the cloves and let the stewed apples cool a bit before eating.

Ayurveda and taste

According to Ayurveda, foods have aromas made up of six separate tastes. Each taste is a combination of the different elements, and has several qualities:

- Sweet (Earth & Water) – increases Kapha. Sweet food is cooling, heavy, and oily
- Salty (Water & Fire) – increases Kapha & Pitta. Salty food is heating and oily
- Sour (Earth & Fire) – increases Pitta & Kapha. Sour food is heating, oily, and light

- Pungent (Fire & Air) – increases Pitta & Vata. Pungent food is heating, dry, and light
- Bitter (Air & Space) – increases Vata. Bitter food is light, cooling, and dry
- Astringent (Air & Earth) – increases Vata. Astringent food is dry, cooling, and heavy

According to the Ayurvedic principles, if you want to balance an elevated Dosha, you need to reduce your intake of the foods that increase that exact Dosha. So if you have an increased Kapha, you should avoid, or cut down on, sweet foods.

Sounds complicated? Don't worry. This connection between your Dosha and the tastes of food is what we will explore in later sections.

But let us end this section in a tasty way: Here is my recipe for **Golden Milk Spice Blend**! You will need:

- 125 ml ground turmeric
- 3 tbsp ground cinnamon
- 2 tsp ground black pepper
- 2 tbsp ground ginger
- 0.5 tsp ground chili

Mix everything together and keep in an airtight container in the cupboard. When you feel like a cup of Golden Milk, stir in 2 teaspoons of Golden Milk Spice Blend in a large cup of warm milk of choice. The Golden Milk Spice Blend is also great stirred into smoothies and yoghurt.

The three Doshas and why different bodies need different food

We have already touched upon the subject of Doshas, or bodily constitutions. But how do we determine what Dosha we have? And did you know that the shape of your teeth, and the colour of your lips, are part of finding your innate constitution in Ayurveda?

Depending on a variety of factors (not only teeth and lips!), we all fit into three main categories of body types: Vata Dosha, Pitta Dosha, and Kapha Dosha.

Prakruti is the name of your innate constitution – the Dosha you inherited from your parents, and was born with. Think of who and how you were before puberty, that is, before the age of 12, approximately. This is your essential nature that will remain constant for life. It determines the distinctive qualities of your mind and body when you are in balance. Knowing your Dosha provides invaluable information that will help you get in touch with your body's inner intelligence.

Vikruti (imbalance) is the way you have been doing or feeling lately – the set of imbalances that you are currently experiencing in the body and mind.

If your Vikruti is something else than your Prakruti Dosha, that is a sign of an imbalance that needs attention.

Find your Prakruti and Vikruti by filling in my free Dosha Quiz. Be sure to fill it in twice, once for your Prakruti and once for your Vikruti. Here is the url:

https://gunnhelenearsky.no/wp-content/uploads/2020/10/Dosha-Quiz.pdf

All three Doshas are present in everyone, but the ratio between them varies a great deal from one person to the next. We will get to that in a moment, but first, here is an overview of the essential nature of each Dosha.

Vata Dosha

A Vata person is usually thin and lanky. They are very mentally and physically active and enjoy creativity, meeting people, and traveling. They enjoy warm, humid weather. Common complaints are cold hands and feet, constipation, dry skin, and cracking joints.

When a Vata person is imbalanced, they are often anxious, ungrounded, find it difficult to stick to a routine, and to complete projects. They might also have insomnia and low immunity. The influence of the Air and Ether elements causes their energy, mood, and appetite to fluctuate. They will often swing from eating heavy foods to ground themselves, to ingesting coffee and sugar to sustain intense activity.

Pitta Dosha

A Pitta person is dominated by the Fire element, which makes them strong, intense, and irritable. They are also influenced by the Water element. A Pitta person is of medium build and endurance, and they have a powerful musculature. Their digestion is strong and they display an intense appetite for food and challenges.

They often have freckled skin that easily reddens in the sun, during exercise, when getting a massage, and when blushing. They are strong willed, and good at doing what they think is right. Both in work and play they show intensity and competitiveness, as they are natural leaders and quick learners. This can make them judgmental or impatient. When a Pitta person is imbalanced, they can experience inflammation, rashes, acne, and loose stools.

Kapha Dosha

The strong framed Kapha person has a tendency to gain weight. They are naturally athletic, as long they are exercising regularly, which many Kapha persons find hard. The influence of the Earth and Water elements makes them innately stable, compassionate, and loyal – a true friend for life. They like doing things methodically, step-by-step, and prefer regular routines.

A Kapha person has a slow metabolism. When they are imbalanced, they often feel unmotivated, stubborn, and complacent, even when change is necessary. Kapha persons often benefit from new environments, people, and occasionally fasting.

Combination Doshas

Most people have one dominating Prakruti Dosha. If you have two of equal size, both will influence you, but in different circumstances. If all three are equal, you are *Tridosha*.

If you have two equal-sized Doshas or are Tridosha (or simply feel like diving deeper into the world of Ayurveda), here is a book I highly recommend you buy and immerse yourself in:

Practical Ayurveda: Find Out Who You Are and What You Need to Bring Balance to Your Life, by Sivananda Yoga Vedanta Centre.

Because each Dosha has its own challenges and possible imbalances, there are separate dietary advice for each Dosha. Imbalances are treated with the *opposite*. That's what we will look at in the following sections.

Vata food

In the previous section you had the opportunity to take a quiz, revealing your Dosha or body/mind constitution. If you haven't already done the quiz, please do so now, before we move on. In this section we look at what a Vata balancing diet should consist of according to Ayurvedic principles. We also look at foods to avoid. We begin by looking at when you should follow a Vata diet.

When to follow a Vata diet

- If you have elevated Vata in your Vikruti
- If your Vata may increase because of your lifestyle
- If you have a strong Vata in your Prakruti
- During late fall and winter, in dry, windy, and cold weather
- In old age

Vata eating habits

Eat sweet, sour, and salty foods to balance out the airy, windy characteristics of Vata. If you don't already have daily meal routines, be sure to set them now so that you can eat regularly. You should also try to eat in a calm and unhurried atmosphere, sitting down. No desktop eating or eating on the run! Because Vata has an inbuilt coolness, you will be surprised to see how choosing warm, cooked foods such as soups and stews will soothe your mind and body. The same goes for beverages, drink hot beverages only.

Vata balancing foods

Let grains be the main part of your food, 55% is recommended for Vata. Use grains such as wheat, white rice, quinoa, spelt, and cooked oats.

Vegetables should make up 20% of your food intake. Use these sweet-tasting varieties: Fennel, cucumber, carrots, squash, spinach, sweet potatoes, and beets.

In order to ground Vata, you need a fair amount of oils from several sources. Therefore it is recommended that fats, dairy, and nuts make up 15% of your food intake. Use ghee (clarified butter) and all oils, except coconut. You can also have salted butter, fresh cheese, heated cow's milk, sour cream, sweet cream, almonds, walnuts, hazelnuts, pumpkin seeds, and sesame seeds.

Your plant proteins is to be found in legumes or pulses, but 10% of your food is enough. Use mung beans, kidney beans, and soy milk.

Add-ons for Vata

Foods often need a little (or a lot) of spices and herbs. Good choices for Vata are fennel, ginger, cinnamon, cumin, turmeric, cloves, and sage. You may also use salt to flavour your cooking, preferably Himalayan rock salt. If you want to sweeten up your food, use pure cane sugar, fruit juice concentrate, or molasses. Fruits that calm Vata Dosha are grapes, pineapple, avocados, figs, oranges, and kiwi. Room tempered apple juice or mango juice is fine, but you should preferably stick to hot drinks, like fennel tea and chamomile tea.

Foods to avoid for Vata

The following foods contain Vata characteristics and will enhance Vata. This isn't good if you want to balance Vata.

- **Grains**: corn, barley, whole grains, crackers, popcorn, puffed rice
- **Vegetables**: kale, Brussels sprouts, broccoli, cauliflower
- **Legumes**: chickpeas, white & black & adzuki beans
- **Dairy**: sheep/buffalo milk/cheese
- **Nuts**: bitter almonds
- **Spices**: chili
- **Drinks**: cold or caffeinated
- **Fruits**: pears, unripe bananas

Pitta food

In a previous section you had the opportunity to take a quiz, revealing your Dosha or body/mind constitution. If you haven't already done the quiz, please do so now, before we move on. In this section we look at what a Pitta balancing diet should consist of according to Ayurvedic principles. We also look at foods to avoid. We begin by looking at when you should follow a Pitta diet.

When to follow a Pitta diet

- If you have elevated Pitta in your Vikruti
- If your Pitta may increase because of your lifestyle
- If you have a strong Pitta in your Prakruti
- During summer and early fall, and in hot and humid weather
- In the tropics

Pitta eating habits

In order to dampen the Fire and Water in Pitta, you should choose to eat sweet, bitter, and astringent foods. The astringent taste is perhaps not very familiar to you, so I'll try to explain. It is cooling, like when you chew on a sugar free mint gum and inhale at the same time. That kind of cooling.

As for a Vata balancing diet, it is very beneficial for you to eat regularly, and preferably four small meals a day. If possible, eat with good friends or family, in a friendly atmosphere.

Pitta often has a lot of excess digestive Fire, and you can eat plenty of fruits (outside of meals), as well as vegetables. This Dosha is the only one in which raw foods and salads are fine.

Pitta balancing foods

Let grains make up the majority of your food, 50% is recommended for Pitta. Use grains such as amaranth, whole grains, spelt, barley, and oats.

Aim for 25% vegetables in your diet. Remember to vary between cooked and raw dishes with eggplant, green leafy vegetables, cabbage, carrots, cucumber, beets, peas, and sweet potatoes.

In order to support the strong and powerful Pitta body, let legumes make up 15% of your food, You can have all types, as long as they are soaked and well cooked.

Fats, dairy, and nuts should make up 10% of your food. Choose buttermilk, unsalted butter, fresh cheese, watered-down cow's milk, and sweet cream. You can also use coconut, soaked and peeled almonds, and sunflower seeds.

Add-ons for pitta

Choose sweet, bitter, and astringent spices and herbs, like basil, curry leaves, cumin, cardamom, mint, peppermint, sage, and rosewater. Experiment with new tastes! Use only small amounts of salt, preferably Himalayan rock salt. The same goes for sweeteners – use small amounts of pure cane sugar, fruit juice concentrate, or fresh honey. Enjoy fruits like red grapes, sweet apples, avocados, bananas, figs, pears, and raisins. And when you need a drink, choose from apple juice, mango juice, vegetable juice, fennel tea, jasmine tea, almond, and rice milk.

Foods to avoid for Pitta

These foods contain Pitta characteristics and will enhance Pitta, and that works against the purpose if you want to balance Pitta.

- **Grains**: rye
- **Vegetables**: raw tomatoes, seaweed

- **Legumes**: chickpeas, white & black & adzuki beans
- **Dairy**: yogurt, hard, spicy/blue cheese
- **Nuts**: cashews, peanuts, hazelnuts, walnuts, pine nuts
- **Spices**: chili, mustard, black pepper
- **Drinks**: alcohol, coffee, orange juice
- **Fruits**: strawberries, cranberries, currants, sour cherries

Kapha food

In a previous section you had the opportunity to take a quiz, revealing your Dosha or body/mind constitution. If you haven't already done the quiz, please do so now, before we move on. In this section we look at what a Kapha balancing diet should consist of according to Ayurvedic principles. We also look at foods to avoid. We begin by looking at when you should follow a Kapha diet.

When to follow a Kapha diet

- If you have elevated Kapha in your Vikruti
- If your Kapha may increase because of your lifestyle
- If you have a strong Kapha in your Prakruti
- During spring, and maybe in the cold and wet weather
- In regions with long winters, and much snow, ice, and rain

Kapha eating habits

When you want to balance out the heavy Kapha Dosha, you should eat pungent, bitter, and astringent foods. Eat warm meals regularly, and be sure to eat in a lively atmosphere.

Kapha Dosha is a constitution in which fasting is fine. You can also skip breakfast or dinner without trouble. Be sure to drink hot beverages only, and limit yourself to a maximum of 6 cups per day.

Kapha balancing foods

Because Kapha Dosha is very energy efficient, you should limit your intake of grains to 45%. Use varieties such as millet, corn, buckwheat, rye, and whole wheat.

Enjoy your vegetables! Let them make up 30% of your food. Eggplant, spinach, cauliflower, broccoli, cabbage, kale, spicy and bell peppers, potatoes, and okra are great for you.

For your plant proteins, have some legumes. Let them make up 15% of your food intake. Use varieties such as adzuki beans, peas, yellow and red lentils, mung beans, and chickpeas.

Choose your fats, dairy, and seeds wisely, and let them constitute 10% of your food intake. Olive oil, canola oil, cottage cheese, pumpkin seeds, and sunflower seeds are good for Kapha Dosha.

Add-ons for Kapha

When it comes to spices and herbs, anise, fenugreck, chili flakes, parsley, and nutmeg works well for Kapha Dosha. You can also use moderate amounts of salt, and small amounts of honeydew honey. Enjoy fruits like pineapple, astringent apples, grapefruit, quince, orange, rhubarb, and blueberries.

Always opt for hot beverages of the uplifting kind: ginger tea, chai tea, green tea, and herbal teas with fennel, rosehip, jasmine, chamomile, and/or clove.

Foods to avoid for Kapha

These foods contain Kapha characteristics, and will enhance Kapha – not good if you want to balance Kapha.

- **Grains**: wheat, white flour
- **Vegetables**: avocados, cucumbers, sweet potatoes
- **Legumes**: no restrictions
- **Dairy**: yogurt, hard and spicy/blue cheese, milk, fresh cheese
- **Nuts**: don't eat any
- **Spices**: reduce salt
- **Drinks**: cold drinks
- **Fruits**: avocado, banana, dates, fresh figs, honeydew melon, watermelon

The Sattvic diet

We are now approaching the essence of the Ayurvedic way of eating – the *Sattvic* diet. In this section we look at another way of classifying foods, and how eating more of one type of food – Sattvic – is said to be the ultimate yogic diet.

If you recall what we learned at the beginning of this chapter, you may remember the three *gunas*: *Tamas*, *Rajas*, and *Sattva*. Foods can be sorted into these three categories. We will address all three of them, but let's begin with the ideal – the Sattvic foods.

Sattva and the Sattvic meal

Sattva is the energy of harmony and clarity, and it is the main goal for an Indian guru. The Sattvic diet is believed to help create happiness of mind and to increase purity, strength, health, and joy for those who adhere to the diet.

A sattvic meal is prepared from fresh, natural ingredients (we will come back to exactly which ingredients later). The foods should be eaten freshly cooked, and in moderate amounts, never filling your stomach more than 80%. A sattvic meal is always eaten sitting down, and it is eaten slowly, giving you ample time to chew thoroughly, and savour the flavours and textures. Mindful eating, you may say. The meal is easy to digest, leaving you feeling light afterwards.

Sattvic foods

Include as many of the following foods as possible in your diet. The positive experience of Sattva will lead you to want to refine your tastes, and food choices, further.

- **Whole grains**: Millet, barley, oats, rye, wheat, quinoa
- **Vegetables**: Green leafy vegetables, cucumber, squash
- **Fruits**: Ripe, fresh pears, apples, plums, peaches, figs, avocados
- **Nuts, seeds, legumes**: Moong dal, lentils, chana dal, chickpeas, cashews, almonds, sunflower seeds
- **Dairy**: Fresh milk, ghee, fresh cheese, curd, yogurt (eaten warm and freshly made)
- **Spices**: Turmeric, cumin, coriander, parsley
- **Sweeteners**: Jaggery, honey, molasses

Did you find any unfamiliar ingredients here? Look them up on the internet, or check out your local Asian grocery store. You're in for a treat!

Cut down on Tamasic foods

Tamas is the energy of resistance, and Tamasic foods are thought to make you dull, inert, lazy, and even depressed. These foods are looked upon as stale, decomposed, rotten, or unclean.

Flesh from animals, birds, and fish is out of the question, being that it is dead and rotting. And all kinds of fermented foods are Tamasic – including vinegar, sauerkraut, blue cheese, beer and wine. Overripe fruits are considered rotten. Mushrooms are nature's way of decomposing organic material, and is also thought of as Tamasic. Burnt or barbecued foods are considered unclean, and canned and processed foods, precooked meals, and leftovers are seen as stale.

You can in fact also turn Sattvic foods Tamasic. This happens when you overeat sattvic foods.

Cut down on Rajasic foods

Rajas is the energy of agitation, and Rajasic foods are thought to make you lusty, angry, greedy, selfish, and violent. Rajasic foods are excessively pungent, bitter, sour, salty, dry and burning. Examples are: unripe fruit, chili in excess, caffeine, onions, garlic, radishes, hard cheese, eggs, white sugar, soft drinks, prepared mustards, salty convenience foods, and stimulants like cigarettes.

It is also possible to turn Sattvic foods Rajasic. This happens when Sattvic food is eaten too fast.

Healthy swaps when cooking

If you want to cut down on Tamasic and Rajasic ingredients when you cook your favourite recipes, here are some good substitutes to try out:

- **Meat, fish:** Tofu, tempeh, legumes depending on what dish you're cooking
- **Eggs**: Chickpea flour, tapioca, tofu depending on the effect you want
- **Onions**: Ginger, celery
- **Vinegar**: Lemon juice, lime juice

When is it OK to eat Rajasic and Tamasic foods?

Foods can, and should, be seen as medicine in the Ayurvedic tradition. Therefore, small amounts of Tamasic and Rajasic foods may be used under special circumstances, like an extra powerful drug.

Rajasic foods in moderation can be used medicinally to increase the energy of depressed, or inert, persons. For instance, a spicy chili ginger shot might be just the thing to get you going in the morning.

Tamasic food in moderation can be beneficial in helping to stabilize and ground an overly restless mind. For instance, a busy mother-of-three might need her chicken for dinner to ground and cope.

CHAKRA FOODS

Of all the spiritual practices derived from the East, *Tantra* is the one maybe most misunderstood in the West. Tantra is often perceived as gymnastic sex acts, or endless intercourses. But it is within the Tantric tradition we find the *Chakras*. Patanjali doesn't mention Chakras at all, because Tantra and Patanjali's Yoga Sutras belong to different traditions and philosophical systems.

You may remember that the word *sutra* essentially means strand or thread, a piece of wisdom or knowledge to learn from. Tantra on the other hand, means loom, referring to the loom that weaves all the threads together. Whilst sutras deal with detail and puzzle-solving, Tantra is the expanded mind, the very process of thought itself.

Tantra works with the Chakras, which are subtle energy centres along the central channel of the body. The goal for this chapter is to give you a basic understanding of how we can use food to balance and open our Chakras. And when you have read the chapter you will have a multitude of colourful, and tasty, foods to choose from for each Chakra.

Just to make it clear: While Ayurveda and eating for your Dosha is a complete dietary system that will sustain you, the Chakra balancing foods are not. Rather, they may be seen as add-ons to refine your diet according to your present needs.

This chapter will also be your personal treasure trove of nutritional information on a variety of foods, also useful when planning a diet according to your Dosha.

The Chakra system

In this section we'll look at the Chakra system and the seven main Chakras. We also dive into the field of balancing the Chakra energies with food.

The seven Chakras we will address are the main energy centres of the body. Chakras are considered invisible, and more spiritual, in nature. However, these unseen energy points need to be nourished from physical foods to be sustained, but in moderation.

Chakra translates to wheel in Sanskrit, and you can imagine them like wheels of free-flowing positive energy.

Each Chakra has an exact location in the body. In drawings, they are represented with certain colours, and they are also said to control different aspects of our body and mind.

You may have heard people talk about unblocking their Chakras? This refers to the idea that when all of our Chakras are open, energy can run through them freely. Thus harmony exists between the physical body, mind, and spirit.

Mindfully eating foods of certain colours and qualities is thought to balance and unblock your Chakras.

The root Chakra and its foods

- **Sanskrit name:** *Muladhara*
- **Location:** At the base of the spine, in the tailbone area
- **What it controls:** Survival issues such as shelter, money, and food
- **Balanced vs unbalanced:** When the root Chakra is open, we feel confident in our ability to withstand challenges and stand on our own two feet. An imbalanced root Chakra may cause issues with the legs,

feet, and digestive system, or feelings of not being supported, insecurity, or fear

- **Colour:** Red
- **Foods:** Root vegetables, red foods, brown foods, protein
- **Spices:** Chives, paprika, cayenne

Beets

The beetroot is rich in dietary fibre and folate (a B-vitamin), in addition to being a great source of potassium which regulates our fluid balance. Folate is important for pregnant women as well as for heart health. The main bioactive substances in beets are called betalains, and include betanin and vulgaxanthin. These substances may protect your cholesterol from oxidising, and hence reduce your risk of heart disease.

Potatoes

Potatoes are a great source of potassium, vitamin C and dietary fibres. Potassium will help your fluid balance. Feel free to eat the peel, which is where a lot of the fibres are located. Compared to hot potatoes, cooked and cooled potatoes contain less calories.

Red bell pepper

All bell peppers are packed with vitamin C, but the red one is especially rich in this powerful antioxidant. Did you know that per 100 grams it contains over four times as much vitamin C as oranges do? This isn't the only reason why bell peppers are healthy. They are also a wonderful source of the powerful antioxidant zeaxanthin.

Strawberries

Strawberries also contain more vitamin C than oranges! In addition, they are rich in dietary fibre which will keep your digestive system happy, and are a great source of the B-vitamin folate. The main bioactive substances are anthocyanins and flavonols, which are powerful antioxidants.

Tomatoes

Tomatoes are called man's best friend. This is because they have a high content of the antioxidant lycopene, which is powerful in battling prostate problems. But lycopene is important for your heart health too, so don't skip the tomatoes even though you don't have a prostate. Lycopene is fat soluble, so a drop of olive oil on your tomatoes will increase the absorption of lycopene.

The sacral Chakra and its foods

- **Sanskrit name:** *Swadhistana*
- **Location:** In the lower abdomen, about 2 inches or 5 centimetres below the navel
- **What it controls:** It is associated with all things emotional, sexual, abundant and creative
- **Balanced vs unbalanced:** A balanced second Chakra allows us to express our creativity, form deep, intimate relationships, and pursue our passions. An imbalanced sacral Chakra can lead to commitment issues, stifled creativity, lack of drive, depression, and lower back pain
- **Colour:** Orange
- **Foods:** Omega-3 sources, orange foods, tofu, nuts, seeds
- **Spices:** Cinnamon, vanilla, liquorice

Apricots

The apricot is a low-calorie fruit with a lot of dietary fibre. It is also rich in vitamin E, the youth vitamin that keeps all cells young and healthy. When dried, the water content lowers and this concentrates all the nutrients and the sweetness. Dried apricots are therefore rich in beta carotene, even though the fresh ones cannot claim to be the same.

Carrots

The carrot gets its beautiful orange colour from the pro-vitamin beta carotene, which it is very rich in. Beta carotene is a powerful antioxidant which can prevent various cancers and eye diseases, and strengthen our immune system. There is also a lot of dietary fibre in carrot, and it is both low-fat and low-calorie.

Oranges

The orange contains a number of different bioactive substances that have a powerful anti-aging effect. In combination with vitamin C, these substances become extra effective against premature aging. One of these is hesperidin, which is effective in lowering blood pressure as well as cholesterol levels. It also seems to be anti-inflammatory.

Sweet potatoes

Like the carrot, the sweet potato is high in beta-carotene. Eating more beta-carotene than you need will lend a beautiful suntanned colour to your skin. Even though the sweet potato is sweet, it has a lower effect on your blood sugar levels than equal amounts of potato. The reason is a special bioactive substance found in the sweet potato. Always eat your sweet potato cooked, though – raw sweet potato contains small amounts of hydrocyanic acid.

Walnuts

Walnuts are crammed with nutrition: they are rich in polyunsaturated fats (omega-3), thiamine, B6, folate, magnesium, copper, phosphorus and dietary fibre. And then they are a source of iron, potassium and zinc. Wow – they are like little multivitamin pills, only tastier! The magnesium will help lessen nightly leg cramps. And copper contributes to the normal functioning of your nervous system.

The solar plexus Chakra and its foods

- **Sanskrit name:** *Manipura*
- **Location:** Upper abdomen in the stomach area
- **What it controls:** Self-worth, self-confidence, and self-esteem
- **Balanced vs unbalanced:** A balanced third Chakra will translate into feelings of inner peace, confidence, and self-control. An imbalanced third Chakra can cause feelings of insecurity and lack of purpose, as well as stomach issues
- **Colour:** Yellow
- **Foods:** Whole grains, dairy, yellow foods
- **Spices:** Ginger, mints, turmeric, cumin, fennel

Bananas

The banana is a source of dietary fibre - the greener it is, the more dietary fibre (in the form of resistant starch) it contains. In addition, the banana is a great source of potassium and vitamin B6. Vitamin B6 is beneficial for our heart health and energy metabolism, and it keeps us energized and alert.

Corn

Corn is a starchy vegetable that can be milled and used as flour for breads and tortillas. It is also a good source of the B-vitamin folate, as well as the minerals phosphorus and potassium. Phosphorus is, alongside calcium, one of the major components of our bone tissue. Corn is also rich in fibre. The yellow colour is due to lutein and zeaxantin, the two main antioxidants in corn. These are beneficial for our eye health.

Oats

Oats are rich in iron, but it is especially in oatmeal flour that the iron is available. Oats contain a special type of dietary fibre called beta-glucans. These fibres have a cholesterol-lowering effect in addition to protecting us from bacterial infections. In addition, oats contain a group of exciting and readily-available antioxidants, avenanthramides, which prevent heart disease.

Pineapple

Pineapple is naturally rich in vitamin C. This will help increase the iron absorption from other plant foods eaten at the same tame as the pineapple – lentils or whole grains, for instance. In addition, the pineapple has a high dietary fibre content. The main bioactive substance is called bromelain and is a proteolytic (protein-digesting) enzyme. This means that pineapple as a dessert will help you digest a heavy meal.

Spelt

Spelt contains about the same as wheat when it comes to starch, fibre, and vitamins, but it has a slightly higher protein content and slightly more trace elements. The gluten in spelt is weaker than in wheat, therefore many gluten sensitive persons can eat spelt. If you are gluten intolerant or have coeliac disease you cannot eat spelt.

The heart Chakra and its foods

- **Sanskrit name:** *Anahata*
- **Location:** In the centre of chest, just above the heart
- **What it controls:** Love, joy, and inner peace
- **Balanced vs unbalanced:** This Chakra can influence our ability to give and receive love from others as well as ourselves. A blocked heart Chakra means having difficulty fully opening up to people. Also it can cause feelings of unworthiness, heart issues, anxiety, low energy, poor digestion, and anger
- **Colour:** Green
- **Foods:** Green teas, green foods, raw foods
- **Spices:** Basil, thyme, lavender

Avocado

Avocados are naturally rich in healthy fats, both mono- and polyunsaturated. It is also rich in the B-vitamin folate. Folate contributes to a normal psychological function, as well as the formation of blood cells. It is also rich in potassium, and it is a source of dietary fibre, vitamin E, vitamin B6 and the trace element copper.

Broccoli

Broccoli is crammed with a variety of vitamins, minerals and other health-promoting substances, and therefore, many think of broccoli as a superfood. Many of these nutrients are rejuvenating. The colour of the broccoli symbolizes health – the darker the colour, the more of the healthy substances you get! Like the cauliflower, broccoli contains cancer-preventing sulphur compounds.

Green tea

Unlike black tea, green tea is not fermented, and thus the content of catechin antioxidants is higher than in black tea. When you let the tea steep for two to three minutes, up to 80 per cent of the catechins will be released and benefit you. In addition, the antioxidant quercetin is also present in green tea. Two cups of green tea per day has been shown to keep the brain young and active.

Kiwi

The kiwi is rich in vitamin C, which strengthens your immune system after intense physical activity. It will also facilitate your production of collagen, the substance that keeps your joints supple, and your skin firm. Kiwi is a fine source of folate (vitamin B) and potassium. It is also rich in dietary fibre. The main bioactive substance in kiwi is called actinidine, an enzyme that digests protein.

Spinach

Both the colour and taste of spinach tells you that this is a healthy food. Beneath the green colour there are large amounts of orange carotenoids like beta carotene, lutein, and zeaxanthin. These are powerful antioxidants that protect the body from harmful free radicals. They thus retain the resilience of the skin cells so that the skin looks young and healthy, they keep the heart and blood vessels young, and they prevent cancer.

The throat Chakra and its foods

- **Sanskrit name:** *Vishuddha*
- **Location:** In the throat
- **What it controls:** It represents our self-expression, communication, truth and responsibility
- **Balanced vs unbalanced:** An open throat Chakra allows us to express ourselves truly and clearly. When blocked, it will feel like one has trouble finding the words to say how one truly feels
- **Colour:** Blue
- **Foods:** Drinks, tree fruits, sea plants, high water content foods, blue foods
- **Spices:** Peppermint, sage, salt

Blackberries

Because of all the seeds, blackberries are rich in dietary fibres. In addition, they are a fine source of vitamin C and copper. Copper contributes to normal hair and skin pigmentation, and normal iron transportation to all the cells. The main bioactive substances in blackberries are anthocyanins, the same we find in blueberries.

Blueberries

It is not primarily vitamin C that is blueberries' nutritional forte, although they contain a decent amount of this important nutrient as well. The largest group of antioxidants in blueberries is called anthocyanins. Wild blueberries (bilberries) contain twice as much anthocyanins as farmed blueberries, for they are blue all the way through. The anthocyanins prevent damage to cells, connective tissue, and blood vessels. This, in turn, prevents wrinkles, varicose veins, haemorrhoids, peptic ulcers, and several forms of cancer.

Healthy blood vessels in the brain lower the risk of Alzheimer's and dementia.

Coconut water

Coconut water is abundant in electrolytes like potassium, sodium, and magnesium. If you're having an intense sweat session, especially in the summer months, the electrolytes in coconut water can help to regulate fluid balance, prevent dehydration, and even ensure proper muscle function.

Dragon fruit

This fruit is rich in antioxidants like flavonoids, phenolic acid, and betacyanin. These bioactive substances protect your cells from damage by free radicals, molecules that can lead to cancer and premature aging.

Dragon fruit is naturally fat-free, and high in fibres. It makes for a good snack because it can help keep you full for longer between meals.

Watermelon

The watermelon is, as the name says, rich in water. In fact, it contains 92% water! The red colour of the pulp is due to the important plant antioxidant lycopene, the same you find in tomatoes.

Lycopene is great for your prostate, and heart health. Watermelon also contains cucurbitacin E, a plant compound with antioxidant and anti-inflammatory effects. Bitter melon, a relative of watermelon, contains even more cucurbitacin E.

The third-eye Chakra and its foods

- **Sanskrit name:** *Ajna*
- **Location:** On the forehead between our eyes or eyebrows
- **What it controls:** Intuition, imagination, and wisdom
- **Balanced vs unbalanced:** When balanced, the third-eye Chakra allows us to focus, see clearly, and trust our own intuitions. Imbalanced, it can lead to a lack of direction or purpose in our life. It can also cause tension headaches, blurry vision, balance problems, and sleep disturbances
- **Colour:** Indigo
- **Foods:** Caffeine, chocolate, indigo and dark purple foods
- **Spices:** Juniper, mugwort, rosemary

Aubergine

The eggplant or aubergine has a low content of energy, and at the same time, a high content of dietary fibres. Aubergines are rich in antioxidants, specifically nasunin found in aubergine skin – which gives it its purple colour. Nasunin is a potent antioxidant and free radical scavenger and has been found to protect the fats in brain cell membranes.

Cacao nibs

These rich, chocolatey nibs are made from cocoa beans. They are loaded with nutrients and powerful plant compounds, that have been shown to benefit health. They're rich in iron, magnesium, phosphorus, zinc, manganese, and copper. Magnesium is needed for over 300 different enzyme reactions in your body. This mineral is lacking in many people's diets. Cacao nibs are also loaded with antioxidants, including flavonoids, such as epicatechin, catechin, and procyanidins.

Grape juice

New research suggests that red and purple grape juices may provide some of the same heart benefits of red wine. This includes reducing the risk of blood clots, lowering the LDL ("bad") cholesterol, preventing damage to blood vessels in your heart, and help in maintaining a healthy blood pressure. It all has to do with the health-protecting antioxidants, including resveratrol and flavonoids, that blue grapes are loaded with.

Plums

Plums are naturally rich in dietary fibres. A lot of it is found in the skin, so eat the plums with the skin on. They are high in polyphenol antioxidants, which have positive effects on bone health and may help reduce the risk of heart disease and diabetes type 2. This is attributed to how prunes increase your levels of adiponectin, a hormone that plays a role in blood sugar regulation.

Purple cabbage

Purple cabbage, also referred to as red cabbage, belongs to the Brassica genus of plants. Purple cabbage is a good source of sulforaphane, a sulphur-rich compound that forms when raw cabbage is cut or crushed. Sulforaphane is linked to powerful heart health benefits and cancer-fighting properties. Cabbage can cause gas and bloating if you're not used to eating it. Use caraway or cumin seeds to lessen the troubles.

The crown Chakra and fasting

- **Sanskrit name:** *Sahasrara*
- **Location:** The centre point at the crown of the head
- **What it controls:** Inner and outer beauty, spiritual connection
- **Balanced vs unbalanced:** It focuses on seeking wisdom and joy and understanding. It radiates an energy dedicated to peace, faith, trust and gratitude for our lives. An imbalanced crown Chakra can bring about feelings of confusion, disconnection, and insignificance. It also commonly causes disorders of the central nervous system or headaches, depression, and sensitivity to light
- **Colour:** Violet
- **Foods:** Detox, fasting
- **Spices:** Gotu kola, lavender, incense, smudging herbs

According to Ayurveda the crown Chakra can be activated or opened by fasting, flushing out toxins, and detaching from physical desires such as greed. Fasting, and detoxifying, are said to be beneficial for the opening of the crown Chakra as it awakens to the highest form spiritual communication. The crown Chakra is usually not associated with any type of food, although some say white foods will be beneficial.

Fasting quietens the body and mind. Drink plenty of water, and practice daily meditation to fully integrate your spiritual, emotional, and physical health.

From a nutritional point of view, the cleansing effect of fasting is poorly documented (in fact, the liver works better when it has something to work with). Still, it is easy to understand that many feel cleansed after fasting for a day or more. When you don't take in energy in the form of carbohydrates, fats, or protein, your body will have to draw on its fat reserves to make energy for the cells. This leads to a light ketone intoxication in the brain, and you will probably experience clarity, and a spiritual connection.

And this brings us to the final chapter of this book, where we connect the act of eating with mindfulness and awareness.

MINDFUL AND INTUITIVE EATING

Why does mindful and intuitive eating come naturally to a yogi? And how can we use honesty as a guideline?

Occasionally, books pop up that have a very special meaning for me. And some time back, I was lucky enough to find just that — a book about yoga and food. *The yoga of eating* by Charles Eisenstein is a unique, philosophical book, and I wholeheartedly recommend that you read it.

It's not an Ayurvedic book. Or a diet book. And it is not a book with a recipe for how everyone should live and eat. Luckily, since this notion is utopian, I think. This is a book that addresses how our yoga practice makes us more sensitive to what our bodies whisper to us. Not just on the mat, but in everyday life. And, if we listen well, we can hear what our bodies enjoy the most when it comes to the food we eat.

Mindful eating, and intuitive eating, are both useful approaches to eating in a healthy way. It isn't surprising that many think that they're one and the same. The two complement each other, and have significant overlap, but there are some important differences.

Mindful eating is about being present in the eating experience without judging yourself or the foods you eat. Intuitive eating is a broader framework that goes outside the eating experience, encouraging us to actively reject external diet messaging, and change our relationship with food and our body.

Why do we eat?

The most obvious answer here, is because we are hungry. But I know I sometimes choose to eat also when I'm not feeling hungry. Why is that?

More than once, I've found myself reaching for the dark chocolate on occasions when feelings have been running high. Even though this is certainly no cause for self-recrimination, I've also noticed that when I am eating that chocolate, I'm not actually savouring the taste or texture. Rather, I'm eating it out of a misplaced habit of needing comfort.

How come we feel this emotional hunger, or Heart hunger, as Jan Chozen Bays calls it in her book *Mindful Eating*. Bays has identified seven kinds of hunger. Maybe you can relate to them? I know I do.

1. **Eye hunger** – The appearance of food can influence our choices. Take your time and really look at your food, feeling appreciative, before tasting it.

2. **Nose hunger** – Know how hungry you get when you get that whiff of freshly baked bread? Certain aromas can provoke a hunger response. When eating, smell your food and notice any changes in your body, heart or mind.

3. **Mouth hunger** – Meal satisfaction arises when we are aware of what is happening in our mouth. Which flavour and texture does it want? Maybe it's simply thirsty?

4. **Stomach hunger** – Check how your stomach feels before and after you eat, notice the difference when you eat healthy or less healthy foods. Notice when you eat small or large portions. And is it the clock that says you're hungry, or your stomach's sensations?

5. **Cellular hunger** – Factors like the seasons, our age, or how much physical work we do affect your nutrient requirements. Ask your body what it needs, and listen for the answer.

6. **Mind hunger** – What we read, hear, or think about food impacts our choices. When we eat based on the thoughts in our mind, our eating is usually based on worry.

7. **Heart hunger** – What memories come with certain foods? What do we hope that eating the food will make us feel like? When you have heart hunger, try having a small portion of what you crave and really savour it.

So, before you take a bite of that food you crave, ask yourself: Who inside you are hungry?

The yoga of intuitive eating

Through my yoga practice, I have found a way to experience being present. Yoga not only makes me feel good, it offers me the opportunity to practice balance, self-awareness, and inward listening. I can use this both on, and off, the yoga mat.

By feeling bodily sensations on the yoga mat, by adjusting my weight and position to explore a pose, and when stopping at a depth or intensity that feels just right, right now, yoga builds my self-awareness. Sometimes I need to do less in a pose, or come out of it before the other students, or support myself with props. Yoga can require strength and be hard, but I am constantly working towards the feeling of effortless effort. All of these practices on the mat can be seen as metaphors for how I can make unique, individually inspired choices in my food choices. What kinds of food make me feel heavy and tired after a meal? What kinds of food make me feel light and energized after a meal?

The 10 principles of intuitive eating

Intuitive eating has been around for a couple of decades already. It was created by dietitians Evelyn Tribole and Elyse Resch in 1995, when they published the first edition of their book *Intuitive Eating*. It has its basis in their work with patients recovering from eating disorders.

Their 10 principles of intuitive eating focus on breaking down dieting cycles, allowing us to reconnect with the body's natural signals around food. It helps us to make peace with all kinds of foods, and attuning ourselves to inner cues, to help derive satisfaction from eating.

The goal is to achieve true health by combining internal wisdom with external knowledge.

The 10 principles of intuitive eating are:

- Reject the diet mentality. Stop dieting. It's not working for you, and you are not alone in this.
- Honour your hunger. Eat when your body tells you that you're hungry and stop eating when you are full.
- Make peace with food. No foods are off limits. This removes any guilt you might feel about eating them, and it will lessen the temptation.
- Challenge the food police. Be aware of, and challenge, internal negative thoughts that categorise foods as good or bad.
- Respect your fullness. Tune into your hunger levels, and only eat when you are hungry.
- Discover the satisfaction factor. Savour the experience of eating. Don't multitask when eating.
- Cope with your feelings without using food. We often use food to deal with our emotions, but it doesn't resolve the problem.
- Respect your body. Accepting your body at every size will help you to feel better and make food choices that are logical, rather than emotional.
- Exercise – feel the difference. Focus on how the exercise makes you feel, not the calories burnt.
- Honour your health with gentle nutrition. Select meals and snacks that are nutritious, but also satisfying and tasty.

Butterflies: When one thing changes, every-thing changes

You cannot change your diet and expect all else to be the same. In this section we explore how this works and why this is both beneficial and useful to know.

Another way of seeing this, is the butterfly effect. This is the idea that small things can have non-linear impacts on a complex system. The concept is imagined with a butterfly flapping its wings, and causing a typhoon. And even though this example is far-fetched, small events, or changes, can serve as catalysts that act on starting conditions.

My own experience on the yoga mat has led me to a flexitarian lifestyle. This was by no means an expressed goal anywhere along the line. But when I started listening to my body and how it felt, the small changes I made in my diet, were soon followed by more life changing choices – like quitting my job, moving to a different part of the country, and becoming a freelance nutritionist. It stems from my yoga practice, from that inner listening, and finding my fuel for who I am, right now.

If you adopt a monastic diet, but not a monastic lifestyle, you will crave more substantial nourishment. And if you go to a yoga retreat, but keep on eating your hamburgers, your diet will become a burden to you.

So – is it at all possible for all of us to become vegan?

Why veganism isn't for everyone (and that's completely ok!)

Being honest is a key yogic virtue, according to Patanjali. It also means being honest when it comes to listening to your body's signals, regarding the fuel it needs. Not what you *think* you should eat, but what you *really need* to sustain yourself at this stage in your life.

What Tantra teaches us, is that we are all the same, we are one. The oneness, or *Advaita*, means that there is no distinction between body and mind, or between vegans and omnivores. It is all part of the bigger whole. And in that context, some are more suited to being omnivores. Many of us are parents, bankers, politicians, caretakers, or have other tasks in this world, and this may require a non-vegan diet. Of course we can strive to choose our foods form a set of ethical norms – organic, grass-fed, fair trade.

But if we try to separate our diet from who we are in this world, we may experience tension in our lives. This will surface as cravings, aversions, or maybe even physical illness. Eventually this will resolve, either by our diet going back to what really suits our lifestyle, or by us changing the framework of our lives.

For me, a mild version of the latter happened. My whole life changed. But I would never condemn those who can't, or won't make the same change.

It has to come naturally.

Most people who live by extremely strict and limited diets are somehow separate from this world. If our role is to live fully in this physical world, we may need a diet that is denser, more packed with nutrients, more physical. This resembles the Chakra foods we looked at in the previous chapter – choosing foods for the Root Chakra will ground you, and nourish your ability to raise a family, for instance.

The vibrational energies required by a monk studying the holy texts all day, may be very different from those required of us in the regular world. Thus, the menu of a monastery nourishes a different state of being, than does the menu of a take away-stand for commuters.

So unless you choose to live monastic-like, maybe you need the nourishment of this physical world as well.

Health

Another reason some of us cannot live, and thrive, on a vegan diet, is dietary restrictions or pre-existing health conditions. For instance, vitamin A from plant foods (beta carotene), needs to be converted in our body into retinol ("true" vitamin A).

Unless you have the genetic disposition to do this conversion, you will soon develop a serious vitamin A deficiency if you only eat plant foods.

Another, and emerging, field of interest is our microbiome, that is, our unique microbial gut flora. Despite an overall adaptability of the gut microbiome (eating more plant foods will change it), you might nevertheless be stuck with certain features beyond your control. For instance, our gut bacteria produce vitamin K2, a vitamin vital to our skeleton, teeth, insulin sensitivity, and heart health.

Other than this intrinsic production, vitamin K2 is almost only found in animal foods. So if your gut flora is short on vitamin-K2-producing bacteria — whether from genetic factors, environment, or antibiotic usage — and you stop eating animal foods, then your vitamin K2 levels can sink to dismal levels.

Other health related factors that may impact our possibility to thrive on a vegan diet are:

- our ability to produce choline, an essential, but often overlooked, nutrient involved in metabolism, brain health, neurotransmitter synthesis, lipid transport, and methylation
- the amount of amylase you produce, both in your saliva and gut. This amount will determine how well you can digest starch, a nutrient most vegan diets are high in. Some of us have genes that don't allow for large amounts of starch, meaning we will get unruly blood sugar levels, and an increased risk of developing metabolic syndrome

Wealth

If people say they can't afford to go vegan, you might think you misheard. Because we all know vegetables and grains are cheaper than beef, right? Still, this is a valid objection. And those who say they can't afford fresh produce, most often live in so-called food deserts.

A food desert can be defined as an area that has limited access to affordable and nutritious food, in contrast with an area with higher access to supermarkets or vegetable shops with fresh foods. This is called a food oasis.

Food deserts lack suppliers of fresh foods, such as fish, fruits, and vegetables. In America, most food deserts occur in black, and brown, neighbourhoods, and low-income neighbourhoods. White majority communities contain more than four times as many supermarkets, as majority black communities, statistics show. This means that many people do not have the resources to buy, or even obtain, healthy food, let alone choose organic or fair trade food. And if you worry about keeping your power on, going vegan is not a top priority.

There are many reasons why going vegan isn't for everyone. But I think we can all take a more mindful approach to the foods we choose to eat.

Mindfulness and Thich Nhat Hanh on how to eat

Mindful eating is a bit different from intuitive eating, but as a yogi you will have encountered both. Here we look at what the well-known Zen master, and Buddhist monk, Thich Nhat Hanh says regarding eating. But first, let's remind ourselves about what mindfulness is.

Jon Kabat-Zinn, Thich Nhat Hanh's student, and the universally acknowledged Father of Mindfulness in the West, defines mindfulness as *"awareness that arises through paying attention, on purpose, in the present moment, non-judgmentally."*

According to the small and delightful booklet *How to eat* by Thich Nhat Hanh, mindful eating is paying attention to the foods you eat. A bite of an apple might show you the apple seed, the tree, the orchard, the sky, the picker and so on. A whole world is contained in a mindful bite of an apple.

You can also look at mindful eating in this way:

- Allow yourself to become aware of the positive and nurturing opportunities that are available through food selection and preparation, by respecting your inner wisdom
- Use all your senses. Choose to eat food that is both satisfying to you, and nourishing to your body
- Acknowledge your responses to food (your likes, dislikes or neutral) without judgment
- Become aware of your physical hunger, and satiety cues, to guide your decisions to begin and end eating

Mindful eating is about using mindfulness to reach a state of full attention to your experiences, cravings, and physical cues when eating. It is true presence, here and now. In our modern society, eating has become a mindless act, often done in a hurry. We know it takes your brain up to 20 minutes to realize we're full, so eating too fast may become a real problem. By eating mindfully, you restore your attention and slow down, making eating an intentional act instead of an automatic one.

Thich Nhat Hanh encourages us to smile when we eat. When you sit down to eat with friends or family, take your time to look at each person, and smile. When you have finished eating, and your plate is empty, take the opportunity to be thankful for the food you received, and smile again.

Mindfulness lets us become aware of what to consume, and what to leave out, in order to keep our bodies, our minds, and the planet we live on healthy, and not to cause suffering for ourselves or other beings.

CONCLUSION

As I write this conclusion, I am looking forward to wrapping my hands around a cup of steaming hot tea, and drinking it, mindfully.

I hope this book has inspired you to do the same. I am ever so grateful for having you as my reader. It is an absolute honour that you chose my book.

Also, if you enjoyed this book, would you please be so kind to tell your friends – and also, please leave a few positive words on Amazon! It means so much to me.

And PS – don't forget your free book gift!

Here's the url again:

https://gunnhelenearsky.no/wp-content/uploads/2020/10/eBook-recipes-Gunn-Helene-Arsky.pdf

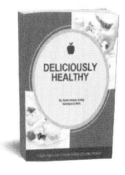

APPENDIX – FOOD AND DRINK BEFORE, DURING, AND AFTER YOGA

Many wonder when, and what, to eat and drink in connection with their yoga practice. Here are my best tips to you, based on science as well as my own experience. But remember: There is no right or wrong way to do this. Listen to your body, and you will know what it needs.

Before class

Traditionally, the physical yoga, your asana practice, is done in the morning, before breakfast. This way you will not be hindered by a full stomach when you turn upside down, and your muscles will receive all the power they need, without blood going to your digestive system. Your mind will also be clear, letting you set an intention for your day.

If your practice is in the evening, many find it useful not to eat anything for the last two or so hours before class begins. Drink a little if you must, or have a light snack an hour before start if you're ravenous.

During class

If you have a regular intensity or strong yoga practice, you would think you may need some extra energy to keep your performance up. Like a banana, or a sports bar. But yoga is not like Zumba, or basketball. You won't need to top up your energy levels unless you're at it for the whole day, in a workshop for instance, and in that case you get a lunch break. Problem solved.

Drinking is another matter. Most yoga teachers will discourage drinking during class. Again, a sloshing stomach full of water may hinder you more than support you. But your yoga teacher has no idea what is going on inside you, so sip some room tempered water if you need to. It is a different matter if you practice hot yoga. Then you're required to bring a water bottle to class, and drink regularly through class. You will sweat a lot, and so you need the fluids.

After class

Unless you have practiced Restorative yoga, you will have worked your muscles to a varying degree during class. While practicing, you use up carbohydrates, protein and liquid. The carbohydrates are stored as glycogen in each muscle cell, and converted into sugar, to give your muscles rapid energy. The protein you use is the very muscle fibres. You actually break down muscle tissue during exercise. The water is lost when you sweat and breathe. Immediately after your practice is over, you must replenish the nutrients you have used up during exercise. This way, your yoga practice will result in a stronger body that is ready for a new practice pretty soon. This is called recovery.

Drink water or tea right after class, and have a light snack containing proteins and carbohydrates, like nuts, a yogurt, or a protein bar. Continue to have small sips of water for the next couple of hours. Then, make sure to eat a more substantial meal within two hours after practice.

CONNECT?

If you would like to connect with me, please visit my Instagram profile and let me know you bought my book: www.instagram.com/gunnhelenearsky

And if you have comments or questions for me, please do email me at yinyangyogaakademiet@gmail.com – I would love to hear from you!

Author profile: www.amazon.com/author/gunnhelenearsky

Online courses: https://www.udemy.com/user/gunn-helene-arsky/

Blog: www.gunnhelenearsky.no

Instagram: www.instagram.com/gunnhelenearsky

ABOUT THE AUTHOR

Gunn Helene Arsky is a Norwegian, holding a Master's degree in nutritional physiology from the University of Oslo, as well as being a Yin and Yang yoga teacher with her own yoga studio in Halden, Norway.

She is a sought-after speaker in Norway, and abroad. She has written a dozen books on nutrition and wellbeing for women, and this is her first eBook. She also writes health and food related articles for Norwegian magazines, and has a holistic wellness coaching practice.

Through these vocations, and her online and offline courses, she helps women to a healthier, happier life, with a green diet and yoga. Food and Yin yoga are her passions, and she is so happy to share them with you!

FURTHER READING MATERIAL

https://en.wikipedia.org/wiki/Patanjali

https://en.wikipedia.org/wiki/Telomere

https://feelgoodeating.com.au/intuitive-eating-and-mindful-eating-whats-the-difference/

https://jivamuktiyoga.com/fotm/magic-cooking/

https://www.acosta.com/news/fresh-meat-and-plant-based-meat-alternatives-on-the-rise-according-to-new-acosta-research

https://www.banyanbotanicals.com/info/Ayurvedic-living/living-Ayurveda/diet/

https://www.cancer.net/navigating-cancer-care/prevention-and-healthy-living/food-and-cancer-risk

https://www.discovermagazine.com/health/what-science-says-about-the-health-benefits-of-plant-based-diets

https://www.health.harvard.edu/staying-healthy/becoming-a-vegetarian

https://www.healthline.com/nutrition/4-reasons-some-do-well-as-vegans#2.-Gut-microbiome-and-vitamin-K2

https://www.healthline.com/nutrition/mindful-eating-guide#rationale

https://www.intuitiveeating.org/10-principles-of-intuitive-eating/

https://www.medicalnewstoday.com/articles/8749

https://www.ncbi.nlm.nih.gov/books/NBK27954/

https://www.ncbi.nlm.nih.gov/pmc/articles/PMC5859346/

Printed in Great Britain
by Amazon

56006927R00043